What's in My Food?

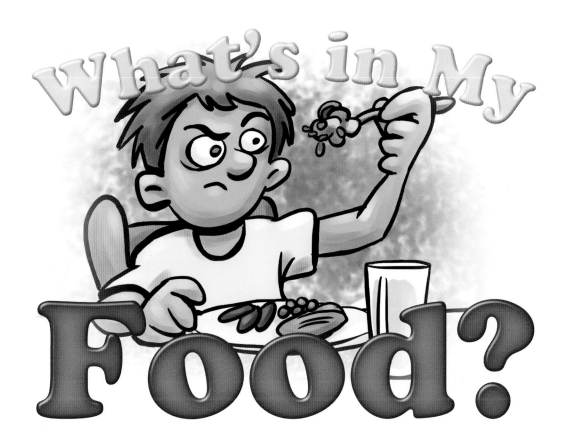

By Deborah Lynn Flores
Illustrated by Ron Wheeler

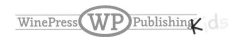
WinePress WP Publishing Kids

For my kids, nieces and nephews—D.L.F.

© 2009 Illustrations by Ron Wheeler.

WinePress Publishing (PO Box 428, Enumclaw, WA 98022) functions only as book publisher. As such, the ultimate design, content, editorial accuracy, and views expressed or implied in this work are those of the author.

ISBN 13: 978-1-57921-953-6
ISBN 10: 1-57921-953-5
Library of Congress Catalog Card Number: 2008920787

Printed in South Korea.

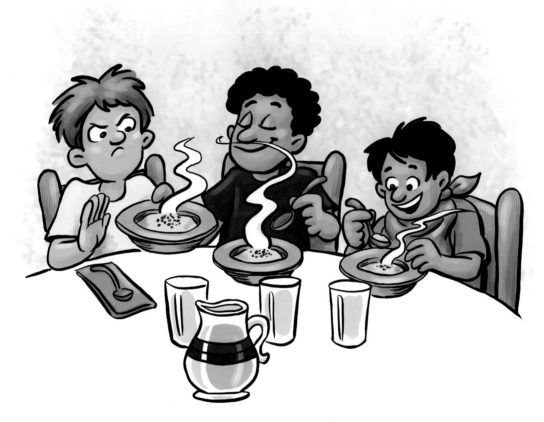

"Cinnamon-raisin oatmeal!" Joseph exclaimed. "My favorite!" The steam tickled his nose. "Eat up," he said, sliding a bowl toward his friend Michael.

"Yeah," Jonah chimed in. "We need energy for our trip today." This was Michael's first visit with the Torrez family, and his first experience with oatmeal. He crinkled his face and pushed the bowl away.

A horn blowing outside soon caught the boys' attention. "It's Mrs. Gibson!" Joseph hollered. Everyone pitched in to clear the table and grab lunches, shouting good-byes and scrambling toward the door.

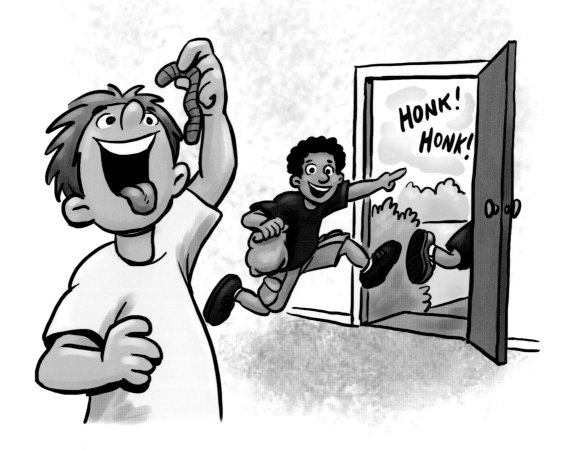

As they hurried to the car, Michael pulled a wiggly jelly worm from his pocket. *Now* **this** *is a yummy breakfast,* he thought to himself. And he ate it.

What do you think of Michael's choice for breakfast? Why don't we eat candy for breakfast?

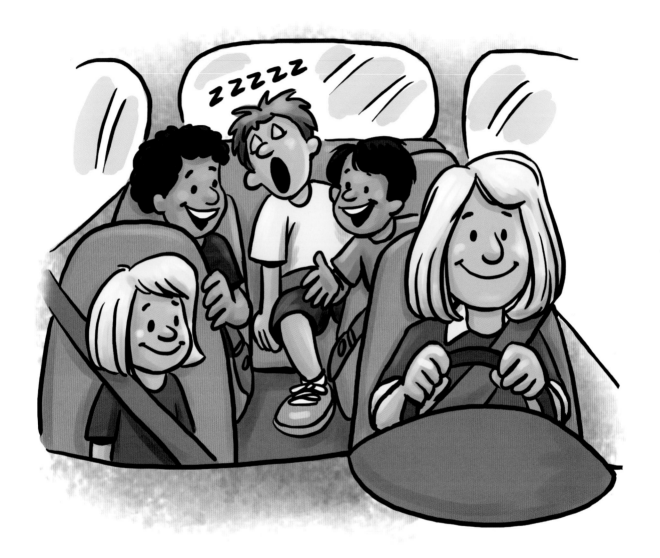

All the way to the theater Jonah and Joseph were full of energy and feeling happy. But Michael leaned his head against the seat. His eyes blinked slowly once . . . then twice . . . and the next thing he knew . . .

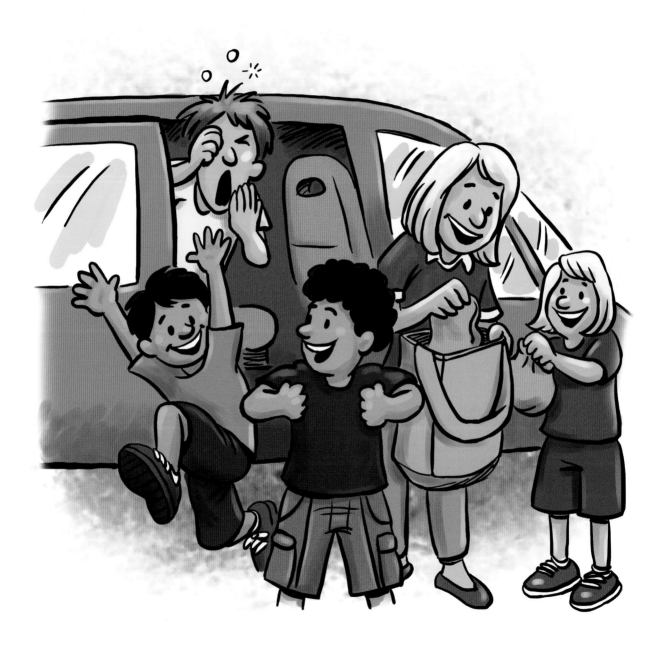

He woke up to find everyone jumping out of the car, excited to see the play, *Peter Rabbit*.

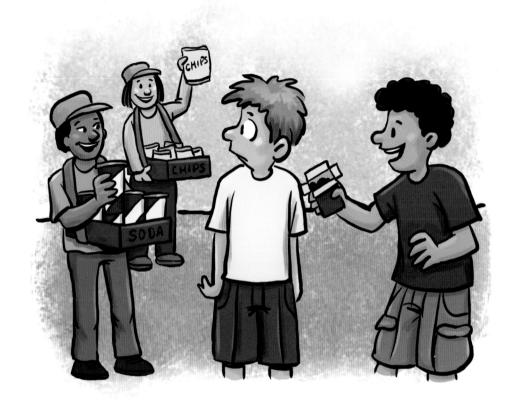

Just inside the theater, Michael's eyes widened. In every corner stood a vendor selling potato chips and soda pop!

"The more fat and sugar you eat," Joseph said, "the worse you will feel. All foods have something your body can use. But when you learn to make better choices, you'll be happier.

"How about some raisins?" Joseph continued. "They have vitamin B." Michael just shook his head and went to his seat.

> There are several different kinds of vitamin B. Some help to fight colds, others strengthen the nerves that tell your brain what you see, touch, taste, and smell.

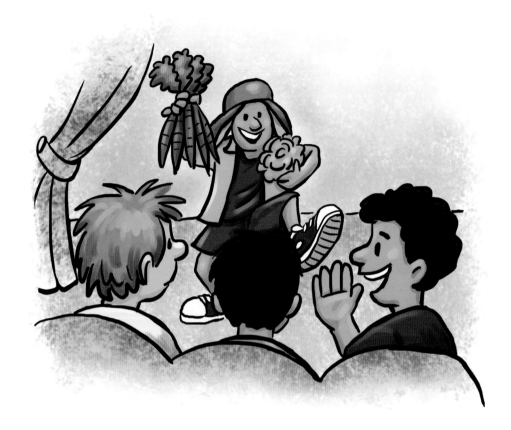

Out onto the stage hopped Peter Rabbit, munching on the biggest bunch of vitamin A, ever! "If I ate that many carrots," Joseph whispered, "my eyes would be so healthy I could see an ant from a mile away."

Jonah giggled and said, "I wonder if Peter Rabbit's mom makes him eat fruits and vegetables five times a day."

"I'm sure she does," Joseph replied. "Most of what a rabbit eats is healthy."

Vitamin A helps keep your eyes, bones, teeth, and heart healthy.

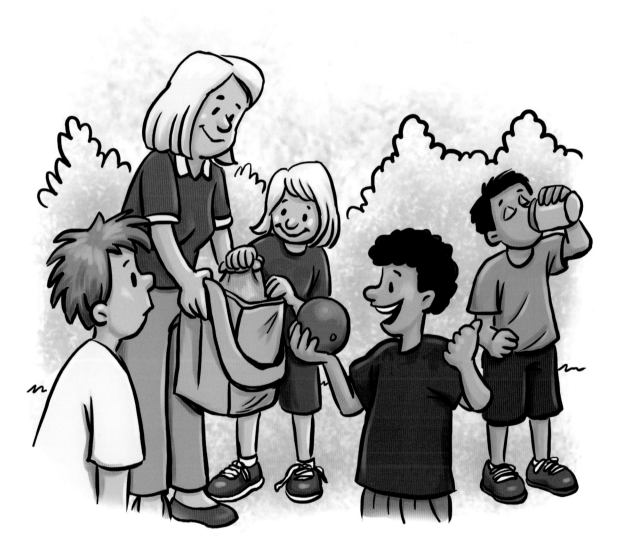

After the show, everyone gathered in the courtyard for lunch. "Mrs. Gibson, did you know that some of the alphabet is hidden in our food?" Joseph asked. "Like the 'C' in this big juicy orange, and the 'D' in Jonah's milk."

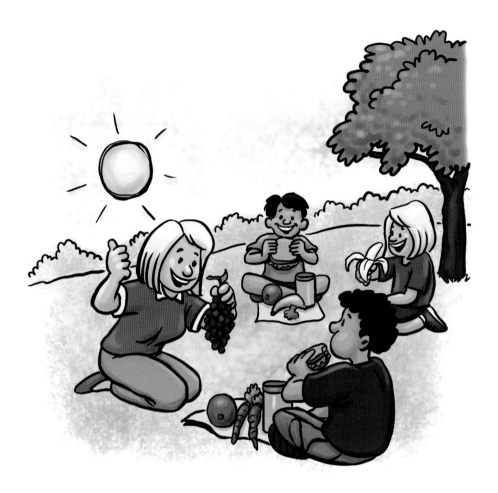

"Did *you* know that all vitamins come from plants or animals?" Mrs. Gibson asked. "There is Vitamin D in milk and other foods. The sun makes the vitamin D work in our bodies to soak up calcium, which makes your bones strong."

It's important to have two to three cups of dairy, or foods with calcium in them, every day.

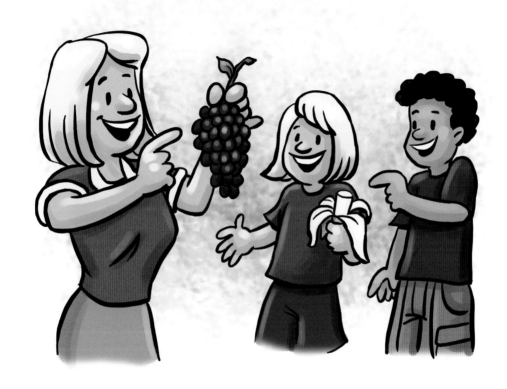

"Wow, Mom, what else can you tell us?" Ally asked.

Mrs. Gibson held up a large bunch of grapes. She smiled and said, "When you eat a grape, you're eating water." A chorus of giggles went through the group. "And, since our bodies are made mostly of water, we need to drink—or eat—lots and *lots* of water!"

"The po-tass-i-*mum* in a banana . . ."

"You mean po-tass-i-*um*," Mrs. Gibson gently interrupted.

"Yes," said Joseph. "Potassium. Potassium helps our bodies keep the right amount of water. Hey, where's Michael?"

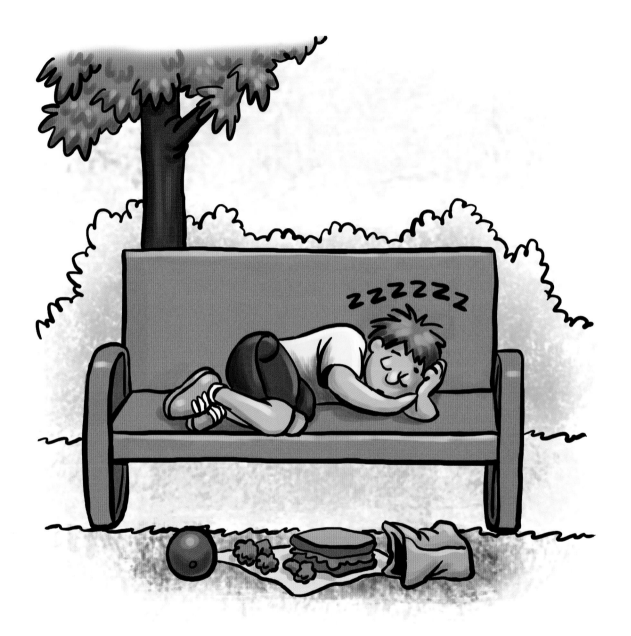

Near a tree in the corner of the courtyard, Michael lay curled up and sound asleep. Beside him, his lunch lay spilled out across the sidewalk—the "A," the "B," even the "C."

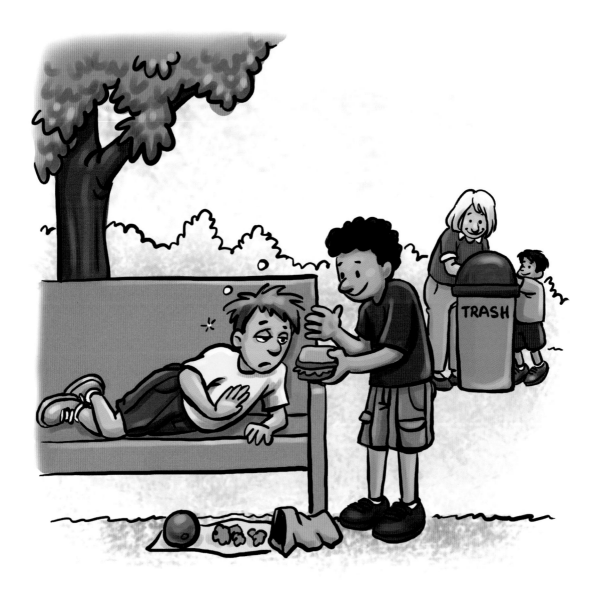

Joseph bent to talk to his friend. "Come on, Michael. You'll have more energy if you eat your sandwich. It's stuffed full of protein."

But all Michael saw was tuna, and he refused to eat it.

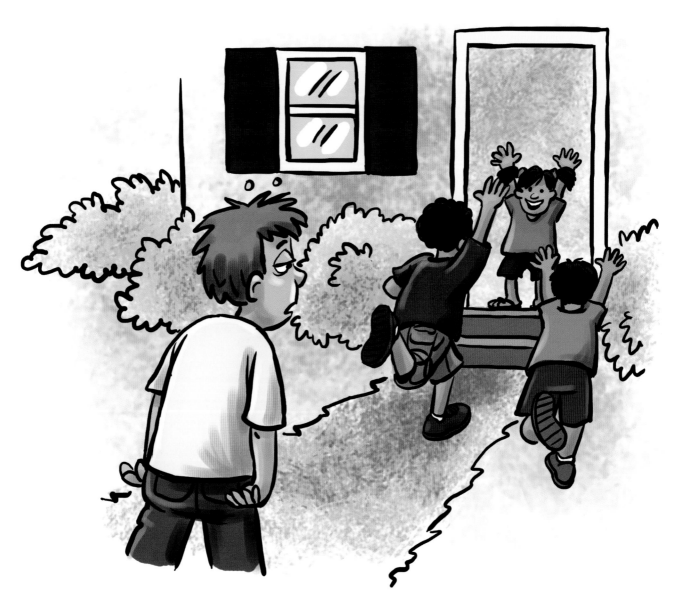

Back at the Torrez house, Mrs. Gibson waved good-bye as Joseph and Jonah raced past Michael. They greeted their sister, Rebekah, and followed her into the kitchen.

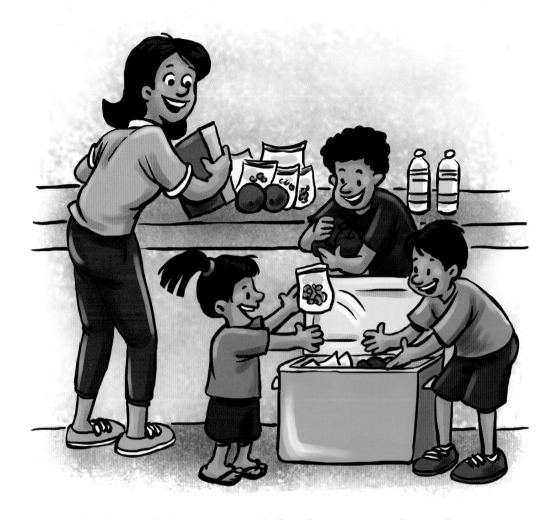

Everyone pitched in to help Mom pack for their trip to the park.
"Watch out!" Jonah teased, tossing a full snack bag Rebekah's way.
"Those cashews might be heavy," Joseph added. "They're packed with iron!"

Iron helps make something your body can't live without: red blood cells.
They take the oxygen you breathe to all the parts of your body.

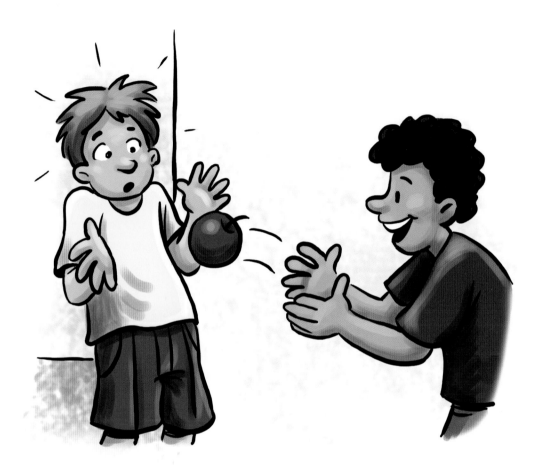

Sleepy Michael came around the corner just in time to catch a fiber-filled apple. "And this big one's for *you*!" Joseph said. "It goes in with the sunflower seeds, walnuts, and water bottles."

Fiber helps your gut stay healthy.
Be careful when buying fruits and vegetables. Many contain dyes and chemicals, particularly on the skins where most of the fiber is found. Some farmers grow organic foods that are not sprayed with chemicals.

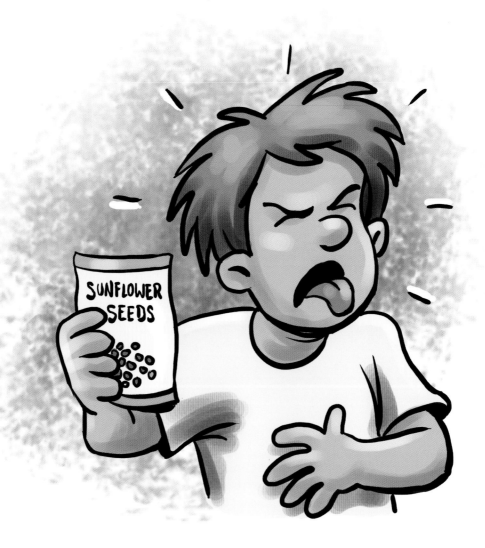

"Sunflower seeds?" Michael made a yucky face.

"Yes," said Jonah. "Mom says that what we eat makes a difference in how our bodies act and feel."

"They have lots of protein, vitamin E, and calcium too," Joseph said. "And they're low in fat!"

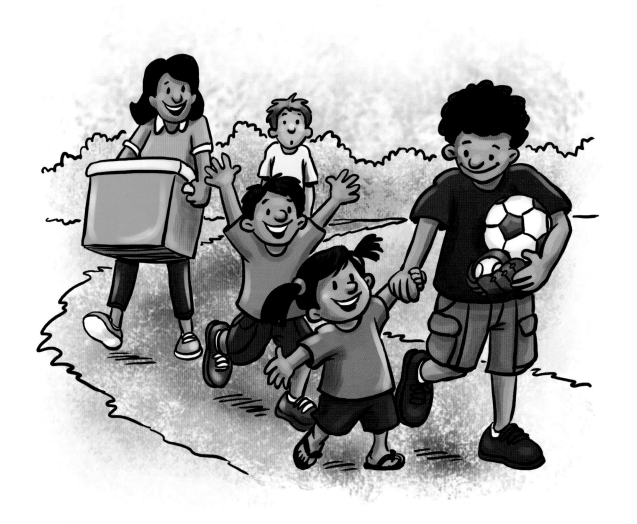

When they got to the park, Joseph grabbed the balls and gloves, took his sister's hand, and headed toward the playground. "Come on!" he shouted. "Our muscles need exercise to grow healthy and strong." Jonah followed while Rebekah toddled along as fast as her short legs could carry her.

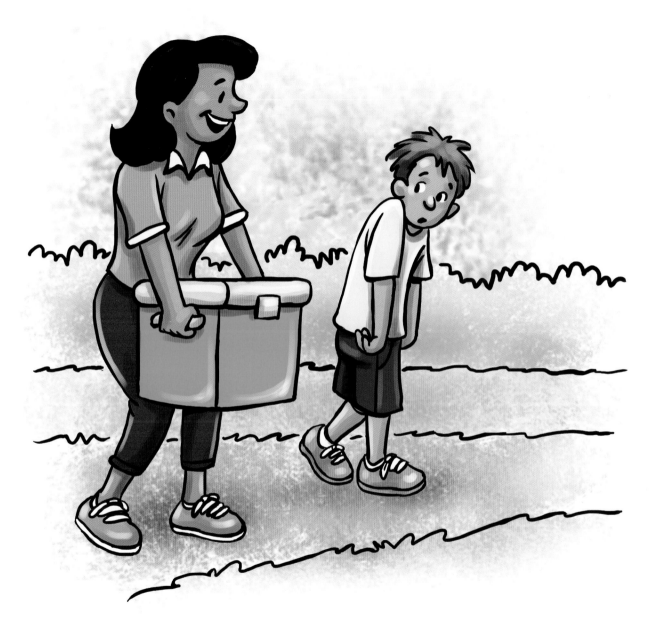

"Go ahead and catch up to them," Mrs. Torrez encouraged Michael. "The run will do your body good."

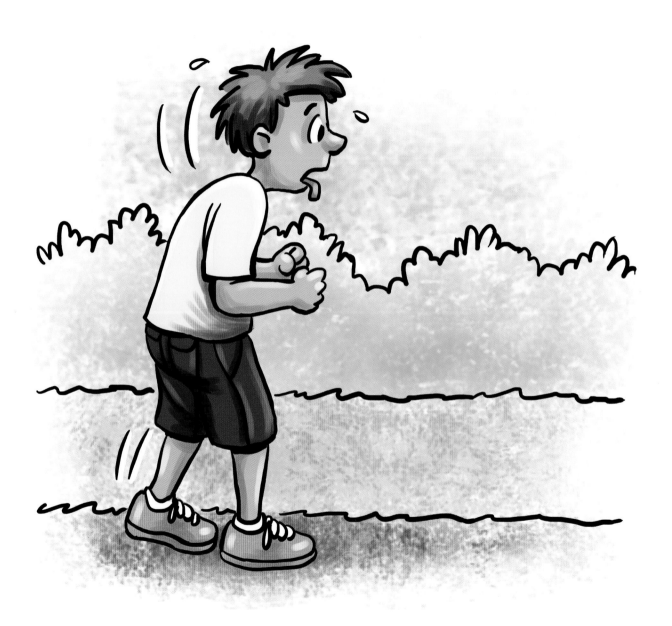

Michael nodded and picked up his pace a little. "Maybe if I had eaten my . . .

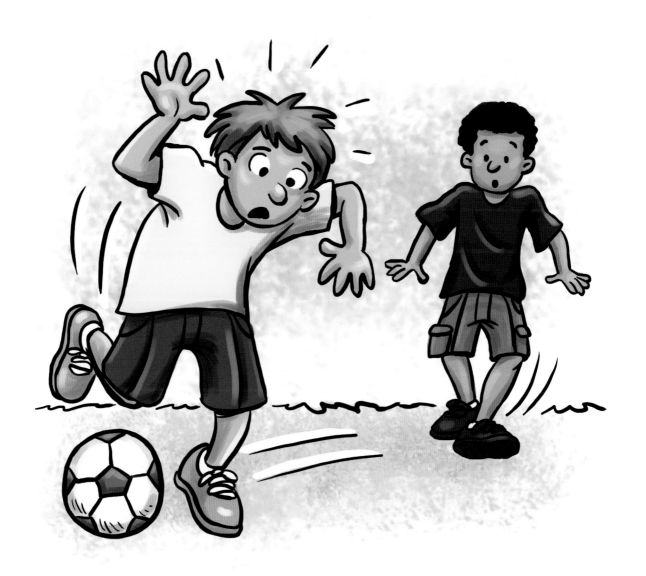

"Yeow!" Michael struggled to keep his balance as a ball suddenly rolled between his feet.

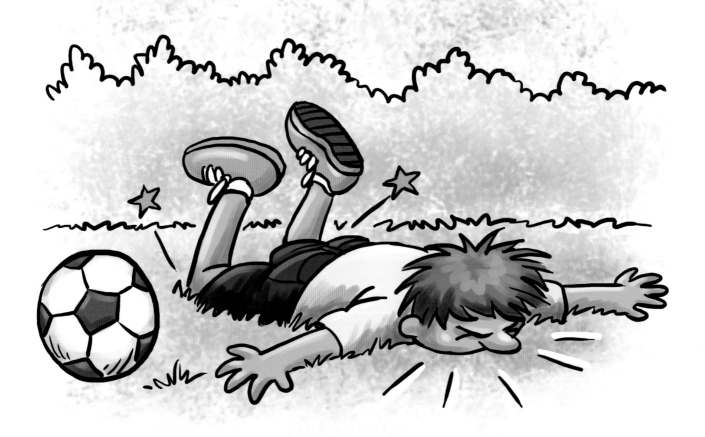

But down he went, skidding on his hands and knees in the tall, prickly grass.

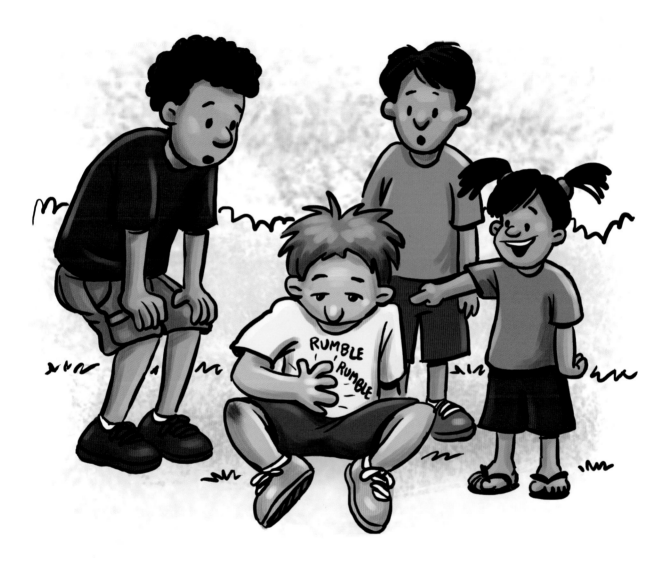

Michael could hardly move. Not because his knee hurt, but because his body was in s-l-o-w m-o-t-i-o-n.

To make things worse, his stomach growled loud enough to wake a sleeping bear, and everyone heard it!

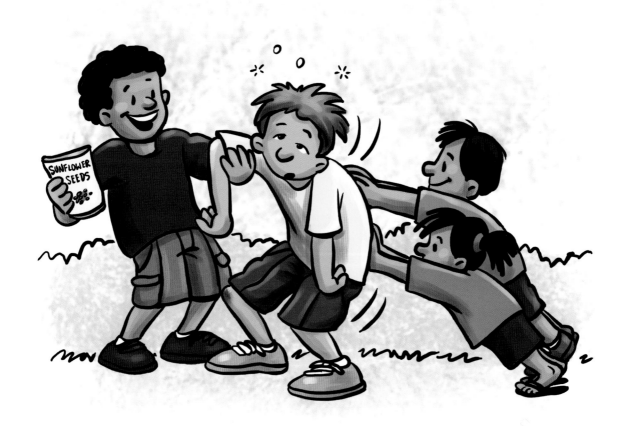

Joseph reached down for his friend's hand while Jonah and Rebekah pushed from behind. "Sorry about that. Here, have some seeds," Joseph offered. "They have good protein and will help you get some strength back."

Michael started to turn his head. Then he remembered that Mrs. Torrez said food makes a difference in how our bodies feel. "OK," he responded. "I'll *try*."

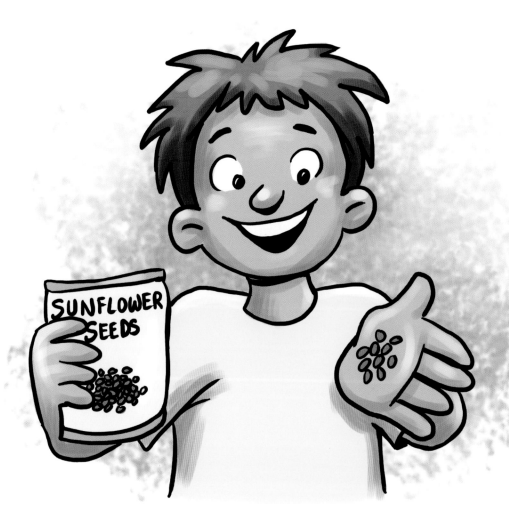

Michael's face lit up. "Hey, why didn't you tell me these were so good?"

Your muscles, hair, skin, blood, and even your brain, all need lots of protein in order to grow strong and healthy.

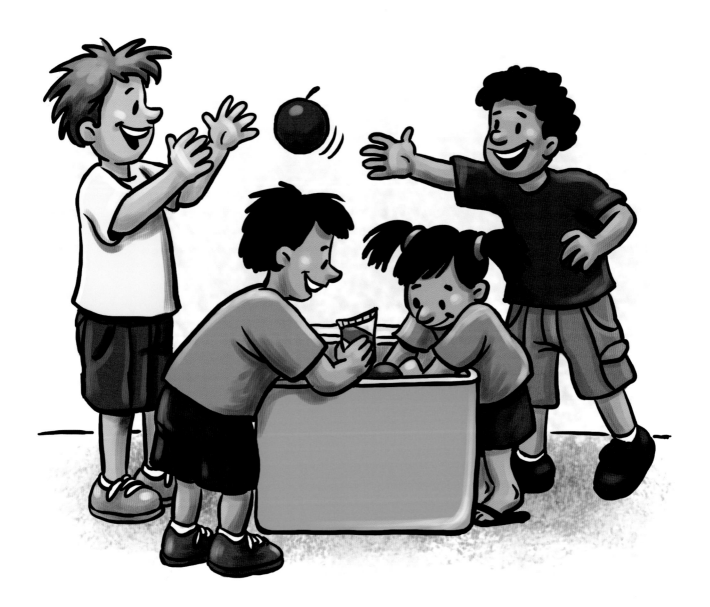

At that, everyone reached into the cooler at once. Michael looked up just in time to catch an apple from Joseph. But *this* time, he didn't grumble. Instead, he sunk his teeth deep into the center of the crispy, red fruit.

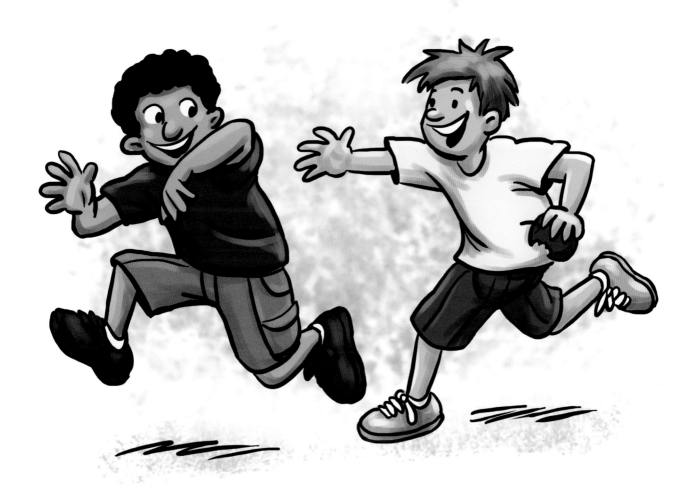

"You're it!" Michael reached out to tag Joseph.

"See what you've been missing all day?" Joseph called out as he took off away from his friend.

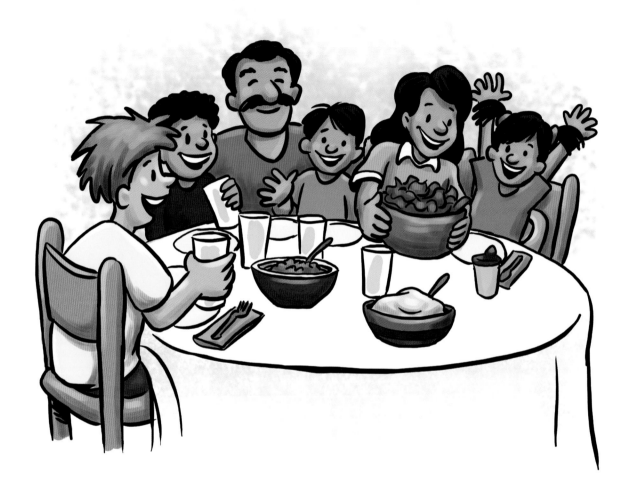

When the family sat down for dinner that night, Rebekah squealed, "Green vitamin K! Michael, it makes your boo-boo all better!" Everyone laughed—even Michael.

When you have a cut, vitamin K helps it to stop bleeding by creating a scab.

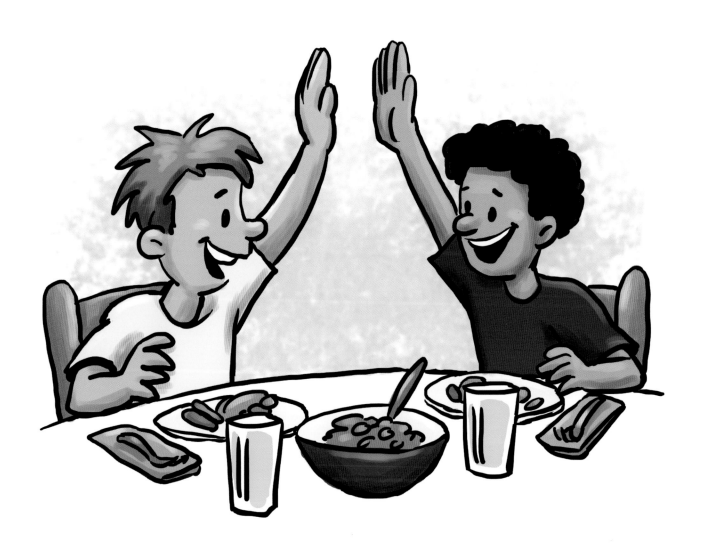

"From now on, I'll make better choices about everything I eat," Michael said. "My body needs more than wiggly worms to work at its best!"

"Way to go!" Joseph cheered. And he reached across the table for the biggest high five of the day!

Parent to Child

- Why were Joseph and Jonah so full of energy and feeling happy on the way to the theater? Let's think of some foods with protein that we can have for breakfast.
- Why was Michael so excited when he first went into the theater? What healthy snacks can you name?
- What happened when Michael didn't eat healthy food? What happens when we do eat healthy food?
- What did Mrs. Gibson tell the kids to drink a lot of every day? What do you drink every day?
- When Michael fell, he scraped his knee. What vitamins help scrapes to heal faster?
- How can we make better choices with the food we eat?

Fresh, whole foods are the best source of the nutrition our bodies need to be healthy. Here's a list to help you start making better choices.

- Vitamin A: Carrots, apricots, broccoli, and other vegetables and fruits that are orange, yellow, and dark green; cheese and fish
- Vitamin B: Red meats, nuts, whole grain foods, and dark green leafy foods
- Vitamin K: Cabbage and spinach
- Iron: Red meat, nuts, eggs, and green leafy foods
- Calcium: Milk, green leafy foods, and fish
- Fiber: Fruits, vegetables, and whole grains
- Water: Berries, table grapes, celery, iceberg lettuce, and cucumbers
- Protein: Eggs, milk, cheese, meats and fish, as well as whole-wheat grains, seeds, nuts, and many other vegetables

* Nuts have a healthy kind of fat and more protein than any other vegetable. Pumpkin and sunflower seeds have less fat than nuts; they also have a lot of iron and calcium.